D-Glucarate™

POWERFUL PROTECTOR AGAINST BREAST & PROSTATE CANCERS

Rita Elkins, M.H.

WOODLAND PUBLISHING
Pleasant Grove, Utah

Woodland Publishing, Inc.
P.O. Box 160
Pleasant Grove, Utah
84062

Contents

Introduction

We live in a time when natural biochemicals and plant nutrients that prompt a wide variety of reactions in the human body are being discovered and studied for their effects as both medicines and preventative agents. In other words, scientists are discovering that putting these compounds in the form of supplements may serve to protect us from health threats more efficiently than we first imagined. D-glucarate™ is such a compound found naturally in some fruits and vegetables. While we know that cultures with diets rich in fruits and vegetables have lower cancer rates, isolating the specific compounds which afford that protection has been extremely challenging. Vitamin C, bioflavonoids, lutein, fiber, indoles and other such nutrients are all found in plant foods and have been isolated as potential cancer fighters. D-glucarate™ now takes its rightful place among these valuable phytonutrients and offers a powerful and unique way to protect our bodies from a myriad of carcinogenic substances we encounter every day. In essence, it expedites the removal of dangerous chemicals from the body, thereby reducing the risk of DNA alteration that can prompt the growth of tumors. Impressive data also supports D-glucarate™'s power to inhibit the formation of cancerous tumors by stopping their proliferation.

Today, more than every before, our exposure to hundreds of cancer-causing chemicals requires an aggressive counter attack to protect ourselves and our families. Certain tissues in the bodies are especially vulnerable to the effects of toxins and harmful hormones. The prostate and the breast are two areas of tissue which can easily bind with chemicals capable of stimulating tumor growth. While men and women are becoming more aware of the valuable role phytonutrients like saw palmetto and soy isoflavones can play, they remain relatively unaware that adding D-glucarate™ to the mix can make it much more effective.

D-glucarate™ ranks high among natural compounds that enhance our ability to rid the body of dangerous substances. Because this compound is not present in sufficient amounts to counteract our exposure to carcinogens, additional supplementation is necessary. Using calcium D-glucarate™ enables the body to do what it can't do on its own: more effectively get rid of cancer-causing substances. In reality, it boosts the body's natural defense system, which in many cases, fails to do the job without help. D-glucarate™ acts as a powerful detoxifier and anti-cancer agent, and because it lacks any toxicity, D-glucarate™ may prove to be profoundly valuable as new cancer preventive compound.

Of equal importance is the ability of D-glucarate™ to lower blood serum cholesterol levels which are directly linked to increased risk of cardiovascular disease. Heart disease and cancer take more lives than any other diseases. Using a safe and natural compound which targets both of these diseases simultaneously is certainly beneficial.

Calcium D-Glucarate™

D-glucarate™, whose chemical name is D-glucaric acid calcium salt tetrahydrate, is a chemical naturally found in fruits and vegetables. The highest concentrations of D-glucarate™ are in apples, grapefruits, broccoli and alfalfa sprouts. This compound exists in two major chemical forms, calcium glucarate and potassium glucarate.

A BRIEF HISTORY OF D-GLUCARATE™

The isolation, purification and use of D-glucarate™ is a patented process and stems back to 1986, when a man named Walaszek and his co-workers discovered that administering D-glucarate™ to both animals and humans resulted in a slow release of a substance that inhibits a chemical called glucuronidase. Glucuronidase is an enzyme that actually blocks the chemical pathway by which the body neutralizes or eliminates cancer-causing substances, also known as carcinogens. This research team found that when animals consumed D-glucarate™, levels of a substance called D-glucaro-lactone became elevated, which inhibited glucuronidase and allowed the body to better rid itself of carcinogens. Walaszek used rats which were given a substance called anthracene. Normally this substance promotes breast cancer development, but he found that if these rats were pre-treated with dietary glucarate, tumor growth was prevented in over seventy percent of the animals.

Of equal interest is the fact that when D-glucarate™ was given to these test animals, estradiol, which is a form of estrogen that can causes breast cancer, dropped. Simply stated, Walaszek discovered that D-glucarate™ has the unique ability to lower the level of glucuronidase, thereby allowing the body to more efficiently eliminate cancer-causing substances it is exposed to. This same team of researchers also found that if they bypassed D-glucarate™ and administered, D-glucaro-lactone orally, glucuronidase activity was reduced for one hour. By contrast, giving calcium D-glucarate™ resulted in a five hour effect.

A number of subsequent experiments were conducted on laboratory test animals which were fed several types of carcinogenic substances. To assess the effectiveness of D-glucarate™, the tests measured their blood levels of free carcinogens (or carcinogens bound to DNA). Test results showed that supplementation with calcium D-glucarate™ significantly reduced these levels over a sustained period of time. Walaszek and his team also concluded that a direct relationship exists between the decrease in the DNA binding of a carcinogen and the ability to induce tumor formation. They discovered that D-glucarate™ actually prompted the expulsion of these carcinogens in the stool, and that this positive effect lasted for several hours after a single low dose.

In 1990, Walaszek moved to the M.D. Anderson Carcinogenesis Center at Houston, and thereafter he published an article reporting that Calcium D-glucarate™ can also initiate a decrease in the proliferation or spread of existing tumors by stunting their growth. During the next three years, subsequent articles appeared that reported test results where D-glucarate™ was actually placed in human tumor cell cultures. In these experiments, Glucarate was added to derivatives of retinoic acid, which is found in vitamin A, resulting in the natural anti-cancer activity of these retinoids potentiated by the addition of D-glucarate™. While the results of this combination were impressive, in 1994, Walaszek demonstrated that used alone, D-glucarate™ was able to stop the growth of certain human tumor cell cultures. Of equal importance is that when tissue cultures had been pre-treated with D-glucarate™, tumor cells failed to grow even when artificially stimulated. In 1995, researchers demonstrated that feeding D-glucarate™ to animals always resulted in its conversion to D-Glucaro-lactone, which subsequently led to increased blood levels of this substance. Again, in the following studies, various carcinogens (N-methyl-N-nitrosurea and others) were administered in order to induce breast cancer in laboratory rats. While the cancer did develop in the rats which were given a placebo, it failed to grow in those animals who had been fed the glucarate.

Additional research by other scientists in 1996 demonstrated that calcium D-glucarate™ and potassium hydrogen D-glucarate™ significantly inhibited colon cancer in laboratory test animals. Other more recent studies have concentrated on the absorption, metabolism, and efficacy of D-glucarate™ in both male and female animals with cancerous tumors. Cancers which responded favorably included breast, prostate, lung, and colon cancer. In each case, the specific mechanism by which these tumors were inhibited remained the same: glucuronidase activity decreased, which resulted in a subsequent lowering of the carcinogen level. In addition, a subsequent decrease in the formation of new tumors was observed.

Dr. Walaszek and co-workers also discovered that dietary D-glucarate™ was able to lower serum cholesterol levels in their test rats. Their results demonstrated that D-glucarate™ and its derivatives were effective in lowering serum cholesterol without increasing cell proliferation and the risk of cancer development. In other words, cholesterol levels went down without any side effects or risks.

In summary, the general consensus reached was that without the help of D-glucarate™, the body's defense mechanisms cannot effectively eliminate cancer-causing agents due to the presence glucuronidase. Supplementation with D-glucarate™ significantly blocks the action of glucuronidase, thus the body can more effectively expel carcinogens, which reduces the risk of lung, breast, prostate, and colon cancers. Moreover, because of its lack of toxicity, D-glucarate™'s potential for lowering cholesterol levels is also an asset.

The majority of the cholesterol research has been conducted at The M.D. Anderson Cancer Center in Houston, Texas. The BioChemix Corporation has continued research in this area using hamster models which correlate more closely to humans, and they are getting impressive results. Full scale human studies are planned for the near future. Simultaneous with the writing of this article, Nutraceutix, Inc. and BioChemix, Inc. have signed a definitive agreement for the exclusive licensing to Nutraceutix of certain patents (U.S. and European) pertaining to the use of glucarate salts and their derivatives for prevention of lung and breast cancer. BioChemix is a technology transfer company whose principals discovered and patented these applications of Glucarate salts at the Science Park of the University of Texas, MD Anderson Cancer Center. Nutraceutix also is acquiring the rights for application of these patents for the prevention of prostate cancer. Selected companies have been licensed to distribute this patented form of D-glucarate™. Through an internationally recognized patent firm, BioChemix continues to secure additional patent protection for its D-glucarate™ technology in the United States and abroad. BioChemix, to date, has been granted the following for D-glucarate™:

U.S. Patent 4,845,123, Cancer Prevention and Use
U.S. Patent 5,364,644, Cholesterol Reduction
U.S. Patent 5,561,160, Anti-Cell Proliferation
(other U.S. Patents are being pursued)
EP 0 528 950 B1, Cholesterol Reduction
(other foreign patents are being pursued)

CHEMICAL ACTIONS

One of D-glucarate's derivatives is a powerful beta-glucuronidase inhibitor called D-Glucaro-1, 4-lactone (1.4-GL). This is the compound that increases detoxification of carcinogens and inhibits tumor proliferation. It blocks beta-glucuronidase by preventing hydrolysis of its glucuronides. 1,4-GL and its precursors may also alter steroid genesis, which is accompanied by changes in the hormonal environment of an effected organ. In a study conducted by Walaszek and published in *Cancer Detection and Prevention*, 1,4-GL was found to be formed from the D-glucarate™ salt in the stomach of rats. Supplemental D-glucarate™ provides a sustained release of D-Glucaro-1,4 lactone (GL) in the digestive tract. It is apparently absorbed from the gastrointestinal tract, transported with the blood to different internal organs, and excreted in the urine and the bile. The formation of 1,4-GL from D-glucaric acid is thought to be required in order to provide protection from chemical carcinogens that could initiate the development of breast, prostate, and colon cancer in humans.

ORGAN-PROTECTIVE PROPERTIES OF D-GLUCARATE™

Through animal studies using a number of different models, D-glucarate™ has been found to have therapeutic actions, including cancer prevention and serum cholesterol reduction. Perhaps its most impressive property is its ability to quickly detoxify the body of chemicals (both artificial and natural) which are potentially harmful. Toxins are neutralized in numerous ways and glucuronidation is one of these. This process involves using the liver to neutralize many chemical carcinogens and steroidal hormones such as estrogen. After a toxin is glucuronidated in the liver, it then goes to the bile and is eventually eliminated in the stool.

The enzyme ß-glucuronidase, which is produced in the gut by unfriendly bacteria, can actually inhibit this process by chemically splitting a glucuronidated toxin before it can be eliminated. This unbound toxin can actually come in contact with the bowel lining and be reabsorbed into the bloodstream, requiring the entire detoxification process to be repeated. When this happens, cells are once again exposed to the chemical, and the liver can become overworked. If D-glucarate™ is present, the troublemaker enzyme is inhibited, and as a result, the process of glucuronidation can proceed without impairment.

What this suggests is that taking D-glucarate™ orally, as a supplement, can provide us with the enhanced and sustained ability to efficiently and rapidly rid ourselves of toxins through unimpeded glucuronidation. In addition, D-glucarate™ does not work like an antioxidant which scavenges or neutralizes damaging structures called free radicals. Instead, it actually forms a type of bond with harmful compounds enhancing their rapid removal from the body. Organs with toxin-sensitive tissue such as the breast, prostate, liver, lung and kidney can especially benefit from this process. These are the organs that can be most damaged by sustained exposure to poisons or carcinogens. In one Japanese study, researchers found that rats who were given kanamycin, a toxic antibiotic, which would normally impair kidney function, were protected if they received D-glucarate™. What they discovered was that the kanamycin was rapidly removed from the body as compared to the non-treated rats. The report stated that, "the drug level in the kidney in non-treated rats was more than two orders of magnitude higher than those in other organs such as the liver, lung and spleen, and remained high for 48 hours after antibiotic administration. In D-glucarate™-treated rats the kidney content of the drug was diminished as compared with non-treated rats just after the antibiotic administration, followed by a gradual decline with time." The positive effects that D-glucarate™ had on test subjects over time is also promising.

PROTECTING OURSELVES AGAINST CANCER-CAUSING CHEMICALS AND HORMONES

The American Cancer Society projected that well over a million new cases of cancer would be diagnosed in 1998 and deaths from cancer would amount to 564,800 people. Because our generation, more than any other, is exposed to a number of potentially harmful environmental pollutants, our contact with carcinogens can reach epidemic proportions. Consider just a partial list of cancer-causing agents and how difficult it is to avoid contact:

- cigarette smoke
- pesticides
- radon
- hormonally-fattened meats
- diagnostic and therapeutic x-rays
- gamma radiation
- trans-fatty acids
- alcohol
- poor diets
- herbicides
- smog
- car exhaust
- certain prescription drugs
- ultra-violet light
- rancid foods
- saturated/hydrogenated fats
- some food/water supplies
- food preservatives
- xeno-estrogens (artificial estrogens in the environment)

While many of us have taken measures to protect ourselves from exposure to the substances listed, we will inevitably and consistently take into our bodies chemicals which can prompt the growth of cancer. Moreover, our own hormones (estrogen and testosterone) can pose a threat if they are not efficiently metabolized and excreted from the body. A new study, partially funded by the National Institutes of Health and the American Cancer Society and published in *Cancer Detection and Prevention*, indicates that Glucarate supplementation amplifies the process by which carcinogens and hormones are removed from the body. In a study published in *Cancer Letter* 1990, Dr. Walaszek talked about the protective potential of D-glucarate™, and how it could exert a positive effect on different stages of the carcinogenic process. He points out that lower cancer rates in some populations may be due to their consumption of food rich in D-glucaric acid, or self-medication with D-glucarate™ alone or in combination with other chemopreventive agents

The protective function of glucarate in the body's natural cancer prevention mechanisms has long been established. Other recent studies indicating the potential use of glucarate in boosting the body's detoxification processes include publications in *Nutrition Research* and *Anticancer Research*. For example, a study published in *Anticancer Research* found that a fifty percent decrease in tumor incidence occurred when glucarate was given to laboratory animals with induced cancer.

Cholesterol Reduction and D-Glucarate™

It is important to stress at this point that more Americans will die of cardiovascular disease in 1999 than cancer. The link between total dietary fat intake and our serum cholesterol levels, along with the risk of developing cardiovascular disease, has been clearly established in recent years. When it comes to cholesterol, what we don't know could hurt us. Cholesterol seems harmless enough. It's nothing but a soft, waxy substance found among other blood fats that helps to build cell membranes and hormones. Circulating cholesterol is a good thing, but a high level of cholesterol in the blood becomes a major marker for a heart attack. Cholesterol and other fats can't dissolve in the blood, so they have to be transported to and from the cells by special carriers called lipoproteins.

Low density lipoproteins (LDLs or least desirable) carry most of our cholesterol through the bloodstream. An excess of LDL carriers can cause cholesterol to accumulate on artery walls (plaque) which supply the heart and brain with oxygen and nutrients. In addition, blood clots can form and lodge in this plaque blocking the flow of blood to heart muscle causing a heart attack. If a clot blocks the flow of blood to any part of the brain, a stroke results. However, LDL is not the only kind of cholesterol, and not all cholesterol is bad. HDL is called good cholesterol because experts believe HDLs carry cholesterol away from the arteries and back to the liver, where it's passed from the body. A high level of HDL cholesterol is preferred, because the higher our HDL levels, the more we are protected against coronary heart disease.

A desirable reading of total cholesterol is less than 200 mg per 100 ml. Borderline readings range from 200 to 239. If you fall into this area, dietary changes and the use of certain supplements may be enough. Anything over 240 is considered high, and may prompt your doctor to advise using cholesterol-lowering drugs.

The ratio of LDL (bad cholesterol) to HDL (good cholesterol) is even more important than the total cholesterol reading. A high risk LDL count is over 160, borderline is from 130 to 159, and desirable levels are less than 130. If you have coronary artery disease, you should keep your LDL levels down to less than 100. Keep in mind that even if your total cholesterol count is acceptable, if you lack in HDL, you may need some dietary adjustments, because HDL readings less than 35 are considered risky.

It is estimated that fifty-one percent of Americans have blood cholesterol values of 200 and higher, and twenty percent have levels of 240 or above. Studies done on people aged 20 and over show that more women have higher blood cholesterol than men after the age of 55, which helps to explain why heart disease becomes more a threat for post-menopausal women. If a person's cholesterol count falls in the range of 200-239, (as it does for over 55 million people), their risk of heart disease is double that of individuals whose cholesterol levels are below 200.

CALCIUM AND POTASSIUM D-GLUCARATE™

Although cholesterol levels directly correlate with heart health, approximately fifty percent of people who survive heart attacks have serum lipid levels in the normal range. What this implies is that other risk factors are involved, including high blood pressure, diabetes, and homocysteine levels. Obesity and diabetes can both increase LDL cholesterol (the bad kind) and decrease HDL (the good kind). While several prescription drugs are available that can effectively lower cholesterol levels, they come with a number of negative side effects including liver damage, and in some cases, they may even prompt the growth of liver tumors.

Calcium D-glucarate™ and potassium D-glucarate™ were both tested to assess their effect on total cholesterol, LDL cholesterol, HDL cholesterol, VLDL cholesterol, and triglycerides. Dr. Walaszek reported that both the calcium and potassium salts of D-glucarate™ were effective in lowering total cholesterol by thirteen to fifteen percent and LDL cholesterol by thirty to thirty-five percent. Because it is difficult to find effective natural cholesterol-lowering compounds, the potential of D-glucarate™ should not be underestimated, especially because it is so safe.

Lung Cancer and D-Glucarate™

The American Cancer Society reported recently that lung cancer is the leading cause of cancer death among both men and women. Since 1987, more women have died each year of lung cancer than breast cancer, which had been the major cause of cancer death in women for the past forty years. In 1999, there will be about 171,600 new cases of lung cancer (94,000 among men and 77,600 among women), and lung cancer will account for about fourteen percent of all new cancers. There will be an estimated 158,900 deaths from lung cancer in 1999 (90,900 among men and 68,000 among women), accounting for twenty-eight percent of all cancer deaths.

Certainly, the most important risk factor here is tobacco smoking. More than eighty percent of lung cancers are thought to be the result of smoking. The longer a person has been smoking and the more packs per day smoked, the greater the risk. If a person stops smoking before a cancer develops, the damaged lung tissue starts to gradually return to normal. Even after ten years however, the ex-smoker's risk still does not equal the lower risk of a person who never smoked, but an ex-smoker's risk is about half the risk of people who continue to smoke. Nonsmokers who breathe in the smoke of others (also called second hand smoke or environmental tobacco smoke) are also at increased risk for lung cancer. A nonsmoker who is married to a smoker has a thirty percent greater risk of developing lung cancer than the spouse of a nonsmoker. In addition to tobacco smoking, exposure to radon and asbestos can also be factors.

Although the best way to prevent lung cancer is not to smoke, people who have smoked and quit should be aware of the role that D-glucarate™ can play in reducing their risk for lung cancer.

EX-SMOKERS AND D-GLUCARATE™

Taking D-glucarate™ may reduce an ex-smokers' risk of developing lung cancer by blocking cancer-causing agents according to recent studies. Thomas J. Slaga, Ph.D., a leading cancer researcher and chair of the Center for Causation and Prevention at the AMC Cancer Research Center in Denver, believes that glucarate supplementation can offer ex-smokers an effective way to reduce their risk for developing lung cancer. He highly recommends using glucarate not only for ex-smokers, but for anyone with an increased risk of developing cancer. Dr. Anderson points out that even if a person stops smoking, their risk of developing lung cancer is higher. He stresses that stopping alone is not enough and recommends stacking the deck in your favor by increasing your consumption of fresh fruits and vegetables and taking D-glucarate™ supplements regularly.

Breast Cancer and D-Glucarate™: The Data

In addition to the instances of lung cancer, approximately 300,000 new cases of breast cancer are diagnosed annually with an additional 150,000 deaths resulting from the disease. In the midst of aggressive cancer research, the numbers are still shocking, and nothing has yet appeared on the medical horizon which looks very promising. Powerful and potentially dangerous drug therapies can often have disappointing results or pose significant health threats of their own.

The simple truth is that we need to consume more phytonutrients in the form of fresh vegetables, fruits, whole grains, legumes and foods like soy to counteract the profoundly damaging effects of, not only our nutrient-poor diets and pollutants, but the negative impact of circulating estrogen and testosterone as well. Taking D-glucarate™ can impressively boost our ability to eliminate chemicals from the body which have the ability to initiate cancerous breast and prostate tumors.

To better understand how D-glucarate™ may prevent breast cancer, it's important to go over the process of estrogen detoxification. Because glucuronidation is directly involved in breaking down estrogen, researchers theorize that boosting the process may help prevent estrogen-stimulated diseases such as breast, cervical and uterine cancers.

THE ESTROGEN COMPONENT

The hormonal workings of a woman's reproductive system can predispose her to developing certain types of cancer, especially breast and uterine. The longer specific estrogen-sensitive tissue is exposed to circulating estrogen, the higher the risk of developing cancer. For example:

- Women who begin their periods early and stop later than the norm have a higher risk of developing breast cancer due to the fact that her tissues have had a longer encounter with estrogen Women are less at risk for developing breast cancer if they go into menopause early, or if they have their ovaries removed surgically which induces an artificial menopause. It must be stressed here, however, that the hormone replacement therapy which usually follows this type of surgery comes with its own set of possible negative side effects.
- A woman who has had few or no pregnancies also has a higher risk of developing breast cancer.
- The older a woman is when she first becomes pregnant, the higher is her risk of developing breast cancer.
- Women who deliver their first child after the age of thirty-five have a threefold higher risk of developing breast cancer than women who bear their first child before the age of eighteen.
- Women who never become pregnant, and women who never menstruate, have a three or four times higher risk of developing cancer, especially breast cancer.
- If a woman had an abortion in the first trimester of her first pregnancy, whether it was spontaneous or induced, she is 2.5 times more likely to develop breast cancer.
- Women with fibrocystic disease can be predisposed to breast cancer.

What these statistics imply is that when certain cells bind with estrogen for extended periods of time, cellular mutation becomes more likely. Estrogen binds with receptors found in breast tissue making the possibility of abnormal cell replication greater. Medical science has been aware of this estrogen problem and over the last ten years has turned to estrogen-blocking drugs like Tamoxifen for women who have had breast cancer or have a high risk of getting it. A report published in the *British Medical Journal* in 1992 stated that while Tamoxifen may work to block estrogen and reduce the risk of breast cancer, it may actually cause other forms of cancer and can have many negative side effects accompanying it. While there are some effective natural anti-estrogens such as soy isoflavones available, D-glucarate™ remains relatively unknown for its ability to metabolize excess estrogen out of the body.

Circulating estrogen is metabolized by the liver where it binds with glucuronic acid and then is transported to the bowel for elimination in the stool. This particular way of ridding the body of potentially dangerous estrogen employs the enzyme process of glucuronidation discussed earlier. This enzyme can split off the gluconoride that has bound to estrogen and free it up to re-circulate through the bloodstream. As we mentioned earlier, when this happens, sensitive tissue is re-exposed to estrogen, and it must be detoxified all over again, putting an added strain on all body systems, especially the liver. This added stress in repeating the detoxification process gives estrogen a better chance to initiate hormonally-induced cancers such as breast and uterine.

If you have an increased risk for breast cancer, this phenomenon is especially undesirable. For men, the same process can occur with forms of testosterone which also stimulates tumor growth in the prostate. A study published in the journal of the American Cancer Institute in 1991 reports that taking D-glucarate™ can help to stop the enzymatic reaction which frees up estrogen and testosterone, thereby preventing their reabsorption. In other words, it promotes the metabolism of estrogen, testosterone and other environmental carcinogens, so that once these toxins are broken down, they can be excreted from the body.

REVERSING BREAST CANCER?

D-glucarate™ may not only work to prevent breast cancer, but has also reversed it in some animal test cases. In such one study published in the *Israeli Journal of Medical Science* in 1995, researchers tested rats which under normal conditions would all develop breast cancer. The findings reported that of those treated with D-glucarate™, only fifty-six percent developed malignancy. Of equal importance is that of that fifty-six percent there were 87.5 percent less tumors per animal than what was normally seen. For every ten tumors the animals would have developed without ingesting the glucarate, they had less than one. This test dramatically illustrates that D-glucarate™ offers significant benefits in both preventing and inhibiting cancerous tumors.

Prostate Cancer Protection for Men

Prostate disease is becoming increasingly common; in fact, the overwhelming consensus is that if a man lives long enough, he will inevitably face prostate problems. Prostate cancer is a leading cause of death among men second only to lung cancer. The chance of having prostate cancer increases rapidly after age fifty. More than eighty percent of all prostate cancers are diagnosed in men over the age of sixty-five. Currently, males between the ages of forty and sixty have a fifty percent risk factor for developing an enlarged prostate, a condition also referred to as BPH (benign prostatic hypertrophy). Ninety percent of men over the age of seventy suffer from BPH.

The American Cancer Society estimates that in 1999 about 179,300 new cases of prostate cancer will be diagnosed in the United States. The American Cancer Society estimates that 37,000 men in the United States will die of this disease during 1999. Prostate cancer accounts for about thirteen percent of male cancer-related deaths.

Studies suggest that men who eat a lot of fat in their diet have a greater chance of developing prostate cancer. Other research indicates that men with a high-fat diet tend to eat fewer fruits and vegetables, less fiber and more dairy products, and that these factors may be responsible for increasing risk, rather than the amount of fat itself. Like the estrogen component for women and breast cancer, a form of testosterone (Dihydrotestosterone, DHT) can also promote the growth of cancerous prostate cells.

While prostate cancer statistics seem rather grim, the good news is that specific natural compounds are available which not only protect the prostate, but effectively treat it as well, making it possible to avoid prescription drugs or surgical intervention, in some cases, of prostate disease. This often means adding D-glucarate™ supplements to prostate health formulas, not only because of the sensitivity prostate tissue has to testosterone, but other potentially carcinogenic agents as well.

WHY IS THE PROSTATE GLAND SO VULNERABLE TO DISEASE?

This walnut-sized male reproductive gland surrounds the urethra which transports urine from the bladder to the end of the penis. Its location explains why when it enlarges, it causes so many problems related to urination. The primary function of the prostate gland is to produce fluids for semen which enhance the survivability of sperm. Due to nature of its tissue makeup, the prostate gland is more prone to toxin accumulation. This is caused in part by slow blood circulation and the fatty tissue makeup of the gland. The fact that blood flow is rather sluggish in the prostate area explains why antibiotic therapy for prostatitis (prostate infection) takes so long to work. It also helps to explain why male hormones and other chemicals can linger in prostate tissue and are more difficult to eliminate from the body.

While no specific studies exist yet on the enhanced elimination of testosterone with D-glucarate™ supplementation, it only stands to reason that boosting the process of glucuronidation should be able to help clear prostate tissue of carcinogenic substances more effectively.

D-Glucarate™: Safety Issues

Human trials have not detected any evidence of calcium D-glucarate™ toxicity, even at very high doses. Several current trials on the cancer-protective effects of calcium D-glucarate™ are testing doses ranging from four to eight grams daily. Because D-glucarate™ speeds the detoxification of hormones and chemicals, a potential side effect could be that blood levels of prescription drugs being taken may decrease and inhibit their reabsorption. Therefore, anyone taking medications should check with a physician before starting D-glucarate™ and shouldn't discontinue use of cholestoral-reducing or similar medicines withouth the approval of a physician.

Forms of D-Glucarate™

D-glucarate™ is available in tablets, capsules and will soon be included in food bars, powdered drinks, etc. It can also be found in formulas designed to target cancer prevention and cardio-health in both short and long term use supplements. Look for the patented version of calcium D-glucarate™ for quality assurance.

RECOMMENDED DOSAGES

Dosages of D-glucarate™ can vary from the normal dose of 200 mg daily to 1500 mg (if you have had cancer). Women who have had breast cancer or men who have had prostate cancer should be eating diets consisting of fresh fruits and vegetables and whole grains. It is preferrable to take this compound with their meals.

Complementary Compounds for Women

SOY ISOFLAVONES

As thousands of women contemplate their risks for developing breast cancer and whether they should take HRT (hormone replacement therapy), understanding the estrogenic properties of soy isoflavones becomes a vitally important issue. Soy became the subject of intense interest after studies surfaced which confirmed that Asian women have markedly lower incidences of estrogen-related diseases and disorders such as breast cancer, PMS, and menopausal miseries. The data is compelling. Asian women have breast cancer rates up to ten times lower than American women. Moreover, soy-eating Japanese women seem much less vulnerable to PMS, and they have no vocabulary word in their language to describe hot flashes.

Why is this? Soy isoflavones have the distinct ability to compete for estrogen on receptor cells. In other words, the body mistakes them for estrogen, and so they are invited to take their place on receptors paradoxically acting as anti-estrogens. Isoflavones actually fool the body into thinking that estrogen has bound with the proper cells, thereby protecting these same cells from contact with real estrogen (for example, breast tissue). Numerous clinical studies (over 1000) clearly indicate that Genistein (the primary soy isoflavone) acts as a desirable weak estrogen in the body.

More and more women of pre-menopausal age seem to be suffering from a phenomenon called estrogen dominance. Estrogen dominance means nothing more that unopposed estrogen or an imbalance between estrogen and progesterone. When estrogen dominates, it binds with more receptor sites in breast and uterine tissue causing heavy or irregular periods, sore tender breasts, water retention, and even bouts with depression. These symptoms can affect premenopausal women of all ages. In addition, having periods but not ovulating (a condition artificially created by birth control pills) can create an estrogen dominance leading to the abnormal buildup of the uterine lining and subsequent menstrual difficulties. Estrogen can also stimulate cellular growth in breast and ovarian tissue, increasing the risk of cancer.

It is easy to see that the less breast tissue is exposed to estrogen, the more protected it will be against the type of cellular mutations that cause the formation of a tumor. Moreover, the role of soy isoflavones for women is also of great value in controlling symptoms of PMS, and easing menopausal miseries like hot flashes. In addition, because soy isoflavones act as phytoestrogens, they can help to prevent osteoporosis. One other value for post-menopausal women is that soy isoflavones also reduce serum cholesterol and can help to lower the risk of heart disease which threatens post-menopausal women.

A study published in a 1997 issue of *Nutrition and Cancer* reported that while Genistein has only 1/1000 the hormonal action of estrogen, it can attach to breast cell receptors and block its contact with the body's potentially dangerous estrogen. Certain pharmaceutical drugs can accomplish the same thing, but they come with all kinds of serious side effects and risks. Moreover, several clinical studies conducted over the last five years support the ability of Genistein to block the action of tyrosine kinase, an enzyme which is thought to stimulate the growth of cancer.

Researchers at Nebraska's Creighton University School of Medicine in Omaha conducted a study which found that soy can also dramatically reduce the movement of cancer cells within the body from one site to another. The first study to test the effects of soy on cancer metastasis concluded that among forty-five soy-fed mice, dietary supplementation of soy protein significantly decreased the incidence of metastasis and the number of tumors that developed. In addition, a recent study published in a 1997 issue of *Free Radical Research* describes Genistein as the most powerful antioxidant isoflavone, followed by daidzein. Antioxidant compounds are considered significant cancer-protective agents. In a study published in 1997, daidzein emerged as a significant immune booster which may reduce the risk of cancer due to its ability to stimulate lymphocyte activity in a way that Genistein alone could not, suggesting that the two compounds should be consumed together.

Clinical studies have found that test subjects with the highest concentrations of isoflavonoids in their urine were protected against both breast and prostate cancer. The profound physiological significance of isoflavones cannot be overly stressed.

Evidence that consuming soy isoflavones early in life affords women extra protection is emerging, especially against environmental estrogenic chemicals. A study conducted at the Comprehensive Cancer Center in Birmingham, Alabama and published in 1998 concluded that exposure to Genistein in the early years (pre-puberty) significantly protects against chemically-induced breast cancer in laboratory animals. Pesticides and other synthetic estrogen-like compounds found in plastics and other such materials are thought to increase the risk of hormonally-stimulated cancers. Hormonally fattened cattle and poultry may also contribute to estrogen-related disorders.

Bone Density and Soy Isoflavones

For older women, declining estrogen can result in the loss of bone density and eventual osteoporosis. In September, researchers at the University of Illinois in Urbana found that soy isoflavones can help to strengthen the bones of the lumbar spine and can also help to prevent the dowager's hump often seen in postmenopausal women with osteoporosis. When 92 mg of soy isoflavones were consumed per day, bone density increased by 2.2 percent over a period of six months. It's important to realize that most women lose two to three percent of bone density in the initial two to three years following menopause, suggesting that the sooner isoflavone consumption is increased, the better.

One of the most serious concerns women have is deciding whether or not to go on HRT. Some data suggests that without it, a women's risk of heart disease escalates. Once again, soy isoflavones seem tailor made in that they target virtually all major health concerns related to menopause. A Japanese study published in 1998 involving close to 5000 test subjects reported that substantial soy consumption strongly correlated to lower cholesterol levels. Moreover, in an 1997 issue of *Fertility and Sterility*, data from a clinical study found that soy isoflavones appear to boost vascular function and protect the heart, suggesting that using soy supplements may be an alternative to HRT for women concerned about their risk of heart attack.

FLAXSEED

A recent article published in *AntiCancer Research* reported that flaxseed can actually reduce breast tumor growth due to its anti-estrogenic properties. This study also concluded that flaxseed can inhibit the growth of estrogen-independent colon tumor cells as well.

Another study conducted at the University of Minnesota reported that flaxseed consumption resulted in a significant increase of estrogen metabolites in the urine of test subjects. What this suggests is that estrogen was being removed more efficiently from the body. In a March,1998 publication of *Cancer Letter*, new data also confirmed that flaxseed can actually lengthen the menstrual cycle which means less estrogen exposure. Flaxseed, like soy isoflavones, are considered non-toxic anti-estrogens that can be used to lower the risk of hormonally-stimulated cancers.

A recent study published in the March 1999 edition of the *American Journal of Clinical Nutrition* stated that flaxseed has the ability to lower LDL cholesterol (the bad kind) in post-menopausal women. Because the risk for heart disease goes up after menopause, using flaxseed to lower the risk of cardiovascular problems is recommended. Moreover, Canadian scientists have discovered that flaxseed not only reduced LDL cholesterol (the bad kind) and raised HDL (the good kind), but actually reduced existing atherosclerosis as well.

LUTEIN

Lutein is a phytonutrient found in dark green vegetables like spinach, collard greens and kale. It has various health benefits some of which include protection from macular degeneration, a leading cause of age-related blindness. A study published in a 1999 edition of *Nutrition and Cancer* reported that lutein increases a specific kind of gene activity which exerts an anti-tumor action in the body in a way that beta-carotene failed to accomplish. Another study conducted at the Department of Nutrition at the Harvard School of Public Health reported that lutein was among those phytonutrients whose consumption was inversely associated with breast cancer risk in premenopausal women. This held particular value for premenopausal women with a family history of breast cancer.

RED CLOVER

Red Clover is considered a phytoestrogenic botanical that also contains isoflavones. It has traditionally been used as a female tonic and possesses some impressive therapeutic credentials. Scientists at the Baker Medical Research Institute in Australia recently reported that the increased cardiovascular risk post-menopausal women face can be reduced by taking red clover. They stated that arterial compliance, which diminishes with menopause, was significantly improved with red clover isoflavones. When our arteries become less compliant, high blood pressure can result and the heart can experience additional strain, thereby increasing the chances of a heart attack. The study strongly suggested that red clover should be investigated for post-menopausal women as a valuable supplement. Moreover, scientists at the Aerone Biotechnology in San Leandro California confirmed that red clover is a phytoestrogen that ranks among the six highest herbs capable of binding to estradiol (bad estrogen).

Complementary Compounds for Men

CERNITIN (EXTRACT OF BEE POLLEN)

This compound has a dual benefit for men in complementing the action of D-glucarate™. It acts to diffuse toxic substances as proven by various studies, and it also inhibits the growth of prostate gland tissue which has value for both BPH (Benign Prostate Hyperplasia) and prostate cancer. Scientists at the Department of Urology at Osaka Municipal Hospital in Japan have recently reported that seventy-nine men with BPH who took cernitin experienced less swelling and better urination. Doctors at Western General Hospital in Edinburgh also reported that laboratory tests with cernitin disclosed that it exerted a specific beneficial effect on prostate cells alone. They concluded that it obviously benefitted hormone-dependent cells which are prone to tumor development. In addition, another study found that cernitin significantly inhibited the absorption of cadmium (a poison) in laboratory test animals. This helps reduce the risk to the prostate tissue which is vulnerable to chemical toxins. Obviously, cernitin, like glucarate, also contributes a protective effect in the body against environmental poisons which can trigger malignant growths.

Long known for its ability to promote stamina, cernitin also works to control blood cholesterol which helps to prevent atherosclerosis. Prostate disorders have also been linked to diets high in saturated fats. A study published in *Atherosclerosis* reported that cernitin significantly lowered serum lipid levels in test animals and may well decrease cholesterol deposits in major arteries. Interestingly, one of the major causes of impotence in men is cholesterol that has deposited in the penile artery. Taking cernitin can not only benefit the prostate and heart, but may also work to help prevent atherosclerotic impotence.

PUMPKIN SEEDS

Pumpkin seeds are a naturally-rich source of zinc, essential fatty acids, carotenoids, and vitamin E, all of which benefit the prostate gland both therapeutically and preventatively. German practitioners have long been using pumpkin seeds for their beneficial therapeutic effect on the prostate gland, and studies have confirmed its effectiveness. Swedish scientists at the Department of Urology at the Karolinska Hospital in Stockholm recently reported that in a randomized, double-blind study, the preparation curbicin, obtained from pumpkin seeds was compared with a placebo in the treatment of symptoms caused by BPH (Benign Prostatic Hyperplasia). Fifty-three patients took part in the study, which was carried out over a three month period. Urinary flow and other such indicators were measured, and all symptoms of an enlarged prostate significantly improved in the treatment group. In addition, no negative side effects were noted.

BETA-SITOSTEROL

Beta-sitosterol is another valuable phytonutrient and is the most common sterol found in plants. As is the case with so many of the compounds I've discussed, scientific data now backs its efficacy for prostate health. In a systematic review conducted in Virginia at the VA Coordinating Center of the Cochrane Collaborative Review Group in Prostatic Disease, researcher found that compared with a placebo, beta-sitosterol improved urinary symptom scores and flow measures for test groups with enlarged prostate glands. In another study recently published in *Nutrition and Cancer*, scientists reported that cancerous tumors in the prostate that were treated for up to seven days with beta-sitosterol decreased their growth by twenty-four percent. Of equal interest is another study published in *Anticancer Research* which stated that beta-sitosterol inhibits the spread of human colon cells through a similar mechanism. German scientists who conducted a multi-centric, placebo-controlled, double-blind clinical trial of beta-sitosterol for the treatment of benign prostatic hyperplasia concluded that test results show that beta-sitosterol is an effective option in the treatment of BPH. While these studies have looked at the medicinal benefits of beta-sitosterol for existing prostate disease, it only stand to reason that its use as a preventative agent is well justified and highly recommended due to its lack of toxicity.

SAW PALMETTO

Clinical evidence validating the use of Saw Palmetto for prostate health is dramatic, to say the very least. This herb, also known as *Serenoa repens*, has undergone extensive study in scientific trials supporting its use as a primary treatment for both short and long term BPH. Statistics have been impressive showing a very high improvement rate in relieving almost every symptom associated with prostate enlargement after only forty-five days of treatment. Saw Palmetto works by inhibiting the production of Dihydrotestosterone (DHT) which can prompt tissue overgrowth in the prostate. Saw Palmetto contains specific fatty acids called steriles which prevent testosterone from binding to prostate gland tissue receptors. It also decreases the production of leukotrienes, which contribute to inflammation.

Studies conducted with over 1000 men concluded that Saw Palmetto accomplished the same action as Proscar (finasteride), the most common prescription drug for prostate disease, but without any negative side effects. The herb promoted the shrinkage of an enlarged prostate gland just as this Proscar, and it also demonstrated impressive anti-inflammatory properties which help to control swelling and pain.

One recent study found that ninety percent of men suffering form BPH experienced noticeable improvement after using this herb for six weeks. Saw Palmetto is usually cited as the herb of choice in the treatment of BPH. Moreover, it can also be used in cases of prostate cancer due to its ability to reduce urine blockage. Some experts believe that Saw Palmetto may be one of the best deterrent compounds to prostate cancer available. In light of this fact, all men should consider taking saw palmetto singly or in an herbal combination long before they experience prostate disease symptoms.

Complementary Compounds for Both Men and Women

CALCIUM CITRATE

Both men and women should supplement their diets with calcium to prevent disorders which can make the body more vulnerable to serious disease. It is vital that every woman makes sure she is getting enough calcium to help prevent osteoporosis. This diseases is linked with bone loss associated with decreased estrogen production in the post-menopausal years. Most women fail to consume the amount of calcium they need through their diet. In addition, men also need to make sure they receive adequate calcium supplementation. Adult non-pregnant women (25 to 50 years) should consume 1,000 milligrams of calcium daily. Pregnant or lactating women need 1,200 milligrams daily. Postmenopausal women taking estrogen supplements require 1,000 milligrams per day, and postmenopausal women *not* taking estrogen supplements need 1,500 milligrams daily. Adult men (25 to 65 years) should get 1,000 milligrams, and all men and women that are older than sixty-five years need 1,500 milligrams daily.

Low intakes of calcium for prolonged periods of time can lead to a calcium deficiency which can result in osteoporosis, loss of the jaw bone (and secondary oral health problems), hypertension, and other disorders. Supplementation with calcium citrate can provide a high amount of elemental calcium. The citrate salt of calcium has been documented to be well-absorbed and utilized by the body. For maximum benefits, don't take calcium with food containing fiber, because fiber significantly interferes with mineral absorption. It is best to take calcium supplements at night on an empty stomach.

CITRUS BIOFLAVONOIDS

Remarkable bioflavonoids found in fruits such as quercitin, hesperidin and naringenin have been accruing impressive scientific credentials as phytonutrients capable of lowering the risk of both cardiovascular disease and cancer. One very recent study published in February of 1999 in *Anticancer Drugs* reported that quercitin was actually able to inhibit the activity of cancer cells in both their growth and proliferation and subsequently described quercitin as a cancer chemopreventive agent. Another study backs up this action and states that flavonoids isolated from citrus were able to suppresses cytokines, which are linked with tumor growth. Scientists at the Department of Biochemistry at the University of Western Ontario in Canada reported that citrus flavonoids are effective inhibitors of estrogen receptor cells in human breast cancer cells. Naringenin and Hesperidin, two citrus bioflavonoids were also cited as having anti-cancer properties. Scientists have concluded that citrus flavonoids are effective inhibitors of human breast cancer cell proliferation in vitro, especially when paired with quercetin, which is widely distributed in many foods. In addition to these properties, other studies have confirmed the ability of citrus bioflavonoids to lower blood serum cholesterol. In a recent study conducted by Italian researchers, hesperidin was able to significantly increase HDL cholesterol (the good kind) and lower LDL (bad kind), total blood fats and triglyceride levels in both normal test animals and those that had high cholesterol counts.

More Tips for Cancer Protection and Cholesterol Control

There are several things you can do to decrease your risk of both cancer and cardiovascular disease. Interestingly, dietary guidelines are almost identical for both. The risks of red meat for both the heart and increasing cancer risk are well-known. This is, at least in part, due to the fact that the bad enzyme that D-glucarate™ blocks is produced more readily when we eat red meat. Today we are advised to eat a predominantly plant-based diet that includes a variety of vegetables, fruits, and grains. A report called *Food, Nutrition and the Prevention of Cancer: A Global Perspective*, concludes that thirty to forty percent of cancers are directly linked to dietary choices. Some good guidelines to follow include:

1. **Choose most of the foods you eat from plant sources**
   - Eat five or more servings of fruits and vegetables each day
   - Eat other foods from plant sources several times each day
2. **Limit your intake of high-fat foods, particularly from animal sources:**
   - Choose foods low in fat
   - Limit consumption of meats, especially high-fat meats
3. **Be physically active and achieve and maintain a healthy weight:**
   - Exercose for thirty minutes or more on most days of the week
   - Stay within your healthy weight range
4. **Limit consumption of alcoholic beverages, if you drink at all**
5. **Use olive oil for cooking and dressings and don't eat hardened margerines which contain trans-fatty acids.**

NOTE: For every ten pounds of fat you carry, you make 100 mg of cholesterol daily. One of the best things you can do is to eat more fiber. A 1999 study confirms again that adding wheat fiber to your diet can protect you from heart disease by lowering blood fats. It's also great for losing weight.

Why Supplementation of D-glucarate™ and Other Nutrients is Necessary

Only nine percent of our population eats enough fruits and vegetables on a consistent basis. Unquestionably, most of us are not getting enough vitamin C and flavonoid compounds from our diets, not to mention D-glucarate™. In addition, it's important to remember that modern farming techniques, premature harvesting of fruits and vegetables, soil depletion, indefinite cold storage, freezing, canning and cooking may denature food of its vitamin C and bioflavonoid content. Because we know that diseases are often nothing more than nutritional deficiencies, we must make adequate supplementation a priority if we want to enhance our longevity.

References

Abbou-Issa, H.M., Duruibe, V.A., Minton, J.P., Larroya, S., Dwivedi, C., and Webb, T.E., Putative metabolites derived from dietary combinations of calcium glucarate and N-(4hydroxypheny)retinamide act synergistically to inhibit the induction of rat mammary rumors by 7,12-dimethylbenz[a]-anthracene, 1988, *Proc. Natl. Acad. Sci.* USA. 85: 4181-4184.

Abbou-Issa, H., Koolemans-Beynen, A., Minton, J.P. and Webb, T.E., Synergistic interaction between 13-cis-retinoic acid and glucarate: activity against rat mammary tumor induction and MCF-7 cells, 1989, *Biochem. Biophys. Res. Commun.*,163: 1364-1369.

Adlecreutz,C.. H., Soybean phytoestrogen intake and cancer risk, 1995, *Journal of Nutrition*, 125 (3): 757S-770S.

Albertazzi, P. et al., The effect of dietary soy supplementation hot flashes, 1998, *Obstetrics and Gynecology*, 91: 6-11.

Awad AB; von Holtz RL; Cone JP; Fink CS; Chen YC, Beta-Sitosterol inhibits growth of HT-29 human colon cancer cells by activating the sphingomyelin cycle, 1998, *Anticancer Res*, Mar-Apr; 18(2A):1227.

Barnes, S., Rational for the use of genistein containing soy matrices in chemoprevention trails for breast and prostate cancer, 1995, *Journal of Cellular Biochemistry*, 22: 181-87.

Berges, R.R., J. Windeler, et al., Randomized, placebo-controlled, double-blind clinical trail of B-sitosterol in patients with benign prostatic hyperplasia, 1995, *Lancet*, 345: 1529-32.

Bioavailibility of soybean isoflavones dep ends upon gut microflora in women, 1995, *Journal of Nutrition*, 125 (9): 2307-15.

Bio ChemPharmac, 1991;41 (10):1471-7)

Braeckman, J., The extract of *Serenoa repens* in the treatment of benign prostatic hyperplasia: A multi center open study, 1994, *Current Therapy Research*, 55: 776-85.

British Medical Journal, March 28, 1992

Brown, N.M., et al., "Prepubertal genistein treatment modulates TGF-alpha, EGF and EGF-receptor mRNAs and proteins in the rat mammary gland," Department of Pharmacology and Toxicology and the Comprehensive Cancer Center, University of Alabama at Birmingham, *Molecular Cellular Endocrinology* Sept 25, 1998 144(1-2): 149-65.

Burke, G.L., "The potential use of a dietary soy supplement as a post-menopausal hormone replacement therapy," *Second International Symposium on the Role of Soy in Preventing and Treating Chronic Disease*, Sept 15-18, 1996, 21, Brussels, Belgium.

Carbin BE; Larsson B; Lindahl O., Treatment of benign prostatic hyperplasia with phytosterols, 1990, Department of Urology, Karolinska Hospital, Stockholm, Sweden, Br J Urol, Dec;66(6):639-41

Carcinogenesis, 1986;7(9):1463-6

Cassidy A., et al., Biological effects of isoflavones in young women, 1995, *British Journal of Nutrition*, 74 (4): 587-601.

Curley RW Jr; Humphries KA; Koolemans-Beynan A; Abou-Issa H; Webb TE Activity of D-glucarate™ analogues: synergistic antiproliferative effects with retinoid in cultured human mammary tumor cells appear to specifically require the D-glucarate™ structure, 1994, *Life Sci* 54(18):1299-303

DiGiovanni, J., Inhibition of chemical carcinogenesis, 1990, in *Chemical Carcinogenesis and Mutagenesis II*, Cooper, C.S. and Grover, P.L. (eds.), Springer Verlag, Berlin, pp. 159-224.

Dwivedi, C., Oredipe, O.A., Barth, R.F., Downie, A.A. and Webb, T.E., Effects of the experimental chemopreventative agent, glucarate on intestinal carcinogenesis in rats. *Carcinogenesis*, 1989, 10: 1539-1541.

Dwivedi. C., Downie, A.A. and Webb, T.E., Modulation of chemically initiated and promoted skin tumorigenesis in CD-1 mice by dietary glucarate, 1989, J. Environ. Path. Toxicol. Oncol., 9: 253-259.

ElAttar TM; Virji AS, Modulating effect of resveratrol and quercetin on oral cancer cell growth and proliferation, *Anticancer Drugs* 1999 Feb;10(2):187-93.

Furuno K; Matsubara S; Ando K; Suzuki S, Preventive effect of D-glucarate™ against renal damage induced by kanamycin, 1976, J Antibiot (Tokyo), Sep;29(9):950-3

Guthrie N; Carroll KK, Inhibition of mammary cancer by citrus flavonoids, 1998, Department of Biochemistry, University of Western Ontario, London, Canada, *Adv Exp Med Biol* 439:227-36

Habib FK; Ross M; Buck AC; Ebeling L; Lewenstein A., In vitro evaluation of the pollen extract, cernitin T-60, in the regulation of prostate cell growth, 1990, University Department of Surgery (WGH), Western General Hospital, Edinburgh, Br J Urol, Oct;66(4):393-7

Haggans CJ; Hutchins AM; Olson BA; Thomas W; Martini MC; Slavin JL, Effect of flaxseed consumption on urinary estrogen metabolites in postmenopausal women, 1999, *Nutr Cancer* 33(2):188-95

Heerdt, A.S., Young, C.W.., and Borgen, P.I., 1995, Calcium Glucarateas a chemopreventative agent in breast cancer., *Isr. J. Med. Sci.* 31:101-105.

Howaniec M; Mekail A; Chroszcz G., The role of cernitins in cadmium effect on the absorption processes in rat small intestine, *Acta Physiol Pol* 1988 May-Jun;39(3):188-94

Hubbard BK; Koch M; Palmer DR; Babbitt PC; Gerlt JA, Evolution of enzymatic activities in the enolase superfamily: characterization of the (D)-glucarate/galactarate catabolic pathway in Escherichia coli, 1998, *Biochemistry*,

Oct 13;37(41):14369-75
Isr J Med Sci, 1995;31:101-5
J National Cancer Inst, 1989;81:1820-3
Jenkins DJ; Kendall CW; Vidgen E; Agarwal S; Rao AV; Rosenberg RS; Diamandis EP; Novokmet R; Mehling CC; Perera T; Griffin LC; Cunnane SC, Health aspects of partially defatted flaxseed, including effects on serum lipids, oxidative measures, and ex vivo androgen and progestin activity: a controlled crossover trial, 1999, *Am J Clin Nutr*, Mar;69(3):395-402
Klippel KF; Hiltl DM; Schipp B, Department of Urology, Allgemeines Krankenhaus Celle, Academic Hospital, Germany, Br J Urol 1997 Sep;80(3):427-32
Manthey JA; Grohmann K; Montanari A; Ash K; Manthey CL, Polymethoxylated flavones derived from citrus suppress tumor necrosis factor-alpha expression by human monocytes, 1999, *J Nat Prod*, Mar;62(3):441-4.
Minton, J.P., Walaszek, Z., Hanausek-Walaszek, M., and Webb, T.E., B-Glucuronidase levels in patients with fibrocystic breast disease, 1986, *Breast Cancer Res. Treat.*, 8: 217-222.
Monforte MT; Trovato A; Kirjavainen S; Forestieri AM; Galati EM; Lo Curto RB, Biological effects of hesperidin, a Citrus flavonoid. (note II): hypolipidemic activity on experimental hypercholesterolemia in rat, 1995, *Farmaco*, Sep;50(9):595-9
Nestel PJ; Pomeroy S; Kay S; Komesaroff P; Behrsing J; Cameron JD; West L, Isoflavones from red clover improve systemic arterial compliance but not plasma lipids in menopausal women, 1999, *J Clin Endocrinol Metab*, Mar;84(3):895-8.
Orcheson LJ; Rickard SE; Seidl MM; Thompson LU, Flaxseed and its mammalian lignan precursor cause a lengthening or cessation of estrous cycling in rats, 1998, .Department of Nutritional Sciences, Faculty of Medicine, University of Toronto, Ontario, Canada, *Cancer Lett* Mar 13;125(1-2):69-76.
Oredipe, O.A., Barth, R.F., Dwivedi, C. and Webb, T.E., Chemopreventative activity of dietary glucarate on azoxymethane-induced altered hepatic loci in rats, 1989, Res. Commun. Chem. Pathol. *Pharmacol.*, 65: 345-359.
Oredipe, O.A., Barth, R.F., Hanausek-Walaszek, M., Sautins, I., Walaszek, Z. and Webb, T.E. 1987, Effects of an inhibitor of B-glucuronidase on hepatocarcinogenesis. Proc. Am. Assoc. *Cancer Res.*, 28: 156.
Oredipe, O.A., Barth, R.F., Hanausek-Walaszek, M., Sautins, I. Walaszek, Z. and Webb, T.E., Effects of calcium glucarate on the promotion of diethylnitrosamine-initiated altered hepatic loci in rats, 1987, *Cancer. Lett.*, 38, 95-99.
Park JS; Chew BP; Wong TS; Zhang JX; Magnuson NS, Dietary lutein but not astaxanthin or beta-carotene increases pim-1 gene expression in murine lymphocytes, 1999, *Nutr Cancer* 33(2):206-12
Prasad K, Reduction of serum cholesterol and hypercholesterolemic atherosclerosis in rabbits by secoisolariciresinol diglucoside isolated from flaxseed., 1999, *Circulation*, Mar16;99(10): 1355-62.
Res Comm Chem Pathol Pharmacol, Sept. 1986;33:25-32)
Science News, April 25, 1992, 144:266-7
So FV; Guthrie N; Chambers AF; Moussa M; Carroll KK, Inhibition of human breast cancer cell proliferation and delay of mammary tumorigenesis by flavonoids and citrus juices, 1996,Department of Pharmacology and Toxicology, University of Western Ontario, London, Canada.
Nutr Cancer, 26(2):167-81.
Sung MK; Lautens M; Thompson LU, *Anticancer Res* 1998

May-Jun;18(3A):1405-8.

Von Holtz RL; Fink CS; Awad AB, Beta-Sitosterol activates the sphingomyelin cycle and induces apoptosis in LNCaP human prostate cancer cells, 1998, *Nutr Cancer*, 32(1):8-12.

Walaszek, Z., Hanausek, M., Szemraj, J., and Adams, A.K. 1998, D-glucarate™ acid as a prospective tumor marker, *Meth. Mol. Med.*, 14, 487-495.

Walaszek, Z., Szemraj, J., Adams, A.K., and Hanausek, M., Reduced levels of D-Glucaric acid in mammary tumor-bearing hosts and the effect of its supplementation during estrogen replacement and tamoxifin therapy, 1992, Proc. Am. Assoc. *Cancer Res.* 37: 183.

Walaszek, Z. Chemopreventative properties of D-Glucaric acidderivatives, *Cancer Bull* 1993; 45: 453-457.

Walaszek, Z., Szemraj, J., Adams, A.K., Kordari, P., and Hanausek, M., Reduced levels of D-Glucaric acid in mammary tumor-bearing host, 1992, *Breast Cancer Res. Treat.*, 375: 108.

Walaszek, Z., Hanausek, M., Adams, A.K. and Sherman, U., Cholesterol lowering effects of dietary D-glucarate™, 1991, Faseb J., 5: A930.

Walaszek, Z., Hanausek, M., Sherman, U. and Adams, A.K., Antiproliferative effect of dietary glucarate on the Sprague Dawley in rat mammary gland, 1990, *Cancer Lett.* 49: 51-57.

Walaszek, Z., Adams, A.K., Sherman, U., Viaje, A., Rotstein, J.B., Hanausek, M. and Slaga, T.J, Antiproliferate effects of Calcium D-glucarate™ (CG) and D-glucaro-1,4-lactone (GL) on the rat mammary gland, colon and mouse skin, 1990, Proc. Am. Assoc. *Cancer Res.*, 31: 124.

Walaszek, Z., Potential use of D-glucarate™ acid derivatives in cancer prevention, 1990, *Cancer Lett.* 54: 1-8.

Walaszek, Z., Adams, A.K., and Flores, F., Inhibition of 7,12-dimethylbenz(a)-anthracene (DMBA)-induced rat mammarycarcinogenesis by glucarate, 1989, Proc. Am. Assoc. *Cancer Res.*, 30: 170.

Walaszek, Z., Hanausek, M., Sherman, U., Del Rio, M. and Adams, A.K., Effects of (+) glucaric acid derivatives and tamoxifen on human breast cancer cells (MCF-7), 1989, *Breast Cancer Res. Treat.*, 14: 175.

Walaszek, Z., Flores, F. and Adams, A.K., Effect of dietary glucarate on estrogen receptors and growth of 7,12-dimethylbenz[a] anthracene-induced rat mammary carcinomas, 1988, *Breast Cancer Res. Treat.*, 12: 128.

Walaszek, Z., Hanausek-Walaszek, M. and Webb, T.E., Repression by sustained release or glucuronidase inhibitors of chemical carcinogen-mediated induction of a marker oncofetal protein in rodents, 1988, *J. Toxicol. Environ. Health*, 23: 15-27.

Walaszek, Z., Hanausek-Walaszek, M., Minton, J.P. and Webb, T.E, Dietary glucarate as antipromoter of 7,12-dimethylbenz[a]-anthra-cene-induced mammary tumorigenesis, 1986, *Carcinogenesis*, 7:1463-1466.

Walaszek Z; Szemraj J; Narog M; Adams AK; Kilgore J; Sherman U; Hanausek M Metabolism, uptake, and excretion of a D-glucaric acid salt and its potential use in cancer prevention, 1997, *Cancer Detect Prev*, 21(2):178-90

Wilt TJ; MacDonald R; Ishani A, Beta-sitosterol for the treatment of benign prostatic hyperplasia, 1999, The VA Coordinating Center of the Cochrane Collaborative Review Group in

Prostatic Diseases and Urologic Malignancies, and the VISN 13/Minneapolis VA -Center for Chronic Diseases Outcomes Research, Minneapolis, USA, BJU Int, Jun;83(9):976-983

Wojcicki J; Samochowiec L; Bartlomowicz B; Hinek A; Jaworska M;

Gawronska-Szklarz B, Effect of pollen extract on the development of experimental atherosclerosis in rabbits, 1986, *Atherosclerosis*, Oct;62(1):39-45

Yasumoto R; Kawanishi H; Tsujino T; Tsujita M; Nishisaka N; Horii A; Kishimoto T, Clinical evaluation of long-term treatment using cernitin pollen extract in patients with benign prostatic hyperplasia, 1995, Department of Urology and Andrology, Osaka Municipal Juso Citizens' Hospital, Japan, Clin Ther, Jan-Feb;17(1):82-7

Zava DT; Dollbaum CM; Blen M, Estrogen and progestin bioactivity of foods, herbs, and spices, Aeron Biotechnology, San Leandro, California 94577, USA. *Proc Soc Exp Biol Med* 1998 Mar;217(3):369-78

Zhang S; Hunter DJ; Forman MR; Rosner BA; Speizer FE; Colditz GA; Manson JE; Hankinson SE; Willett WC, Dietary carotenoids and vitamins A, C, and E and risk of breast cancer, 1999, Department of Nutrition, Harvard School of Public Health, Boston, MA, J *Natl Cancer Inst*, Mar 17;91(6):547-56.